Osteopathic
Self-Treatment

About the book

The aim of osteopathic treatments is to activate the oftentimes impaired self-healing powers and thereby initiate a completely natural healing. The osteopath achieves this by means of his knowledge of human anatomy and physiology and with finesse of his palpation. The osteopathic techniques are however also wonderfully suited for self-treatment. This is where personal body-awareness comes into play.

In this book, Thomas Seebeck conveys the principles of osteopathic treatment, and particularly the "osteopathic medicine cabinet": exercises for common problem areas (e.g. head, back, sprains) are illustrated in a detailed and practical manner.

About the author

Thomas Seebeck, born 1971, has been a physiotherapist since 1995 and has been running his own clinic in Dinklage (Germany) since 2002. In 2006 he received the Diploma in Osteopathic Therapy from the German Society of Osteopathic Medicine (DGOM), for which he has also been a teacher since 2008. He is the chairman of the German Association for Osteopathic Therapy (DAGOT) and academician of the DGOM.

He dedicates his free time to music, amongst other things, classic Chinese medicine, and QiGong and loves windsurfing. He runs self-awareness courses together with his brother, Andreas.

Thomas Seebeck

Osteopathic Self-Treatment

Finding Health

LOTUS PRESS

Important advice: the methods and suggestions in this book represent the author's opinion and experience. They were compiled according to the best of his knowledge and were tested as carefully as possible. They are not, however, a substitute for competent medical advice. The reader is personally responsible for his actions. Neither the author, nor the publishing company can be held accountable for any negative side effects or damages resulting from following the practical suggestions provided in this book.

Thomas Seebeck
Osteopathic Self-Treatment
Finding Health

Copyright by Lotus-Press, 2014
Layout: Andreas Seebeck

www.lotus-press.com

ISBN 978-3-945430-19-4

For my patients,
who taught me
to "dig deeper".

Contents

*To find health
should be the object of the doctor.
Anyone can find disease.*

A.T. Still

Prologue

"I have asked a few questions pertaining to organic action and life, because Nature is a school of question and answers, which seems to be the only school in which man learns anything."

A.T. Still

What is the secret of the mode of operation of osteopathy?

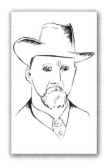

Andrew Taylor Still

When Andrew Taylor Still (1828-1917), the founder of osteopathy, lost three of his then four children to a meningitis epidemic in February 1867, he lost all faith in the conventional medicine of his day.

Still began an intensive study of, what he called, the "Book of Nature". He wondered why his daughter Marusha had survived the illness, and what had made her immune to it. In his study he came across principles that are also known in classic Chinese medicine. Being a technically gifted inventor (of several tools and machines for which he held the patent rights), he viewed the human body as a perfectly constructed machine. Man in his entirety, however, he viewed as a unity made up of body, spirit and soul ("triune man"). From the very start he applied his knowledge and skill not only to his patients, but also to himself.

This book offers you the best methods of self-treatment according to the principles of osteopathy.

Thomas Seebeck, July 2014

Introduction

Sit in an upright and relaxed position on a chair or stool. Take a moment and feel the air flowing through your nostrils.

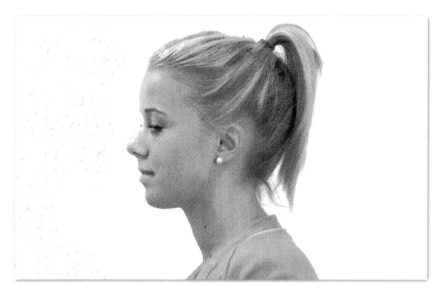

The three components of osteopathic self-treatment: breathing, movement and awareness.

Discern carefully: does more air flow through the right or left nostril or is the difference unnoticeable? Can you feel that the air you breathe out is warmer than the air you breathe in?

Now guide your awareness to your torso and spine. Can you sense that your breathing is connected with a small movement of your torso and spine? When you breathe in, your spine extends a little, and when you breathe out it retracts a little. If you can sense this, then you are ready for your self-treatment, because for this you will not require much more than a sense of breathing and movement.

Your first osteopathic self-treatment

In the introduction I asked you to feel the connection between breathing in and the slight extension of the spine, and breathing out and the slight bending of the spine. Now please try to find out which direction of movement is more comfortable for you. If you cannot be sure with very small movements, simply make the movements larger. Please remember though, that you are trying to find the maximum relaxation. If you move too far into the more comfortable position, the tension increases again.

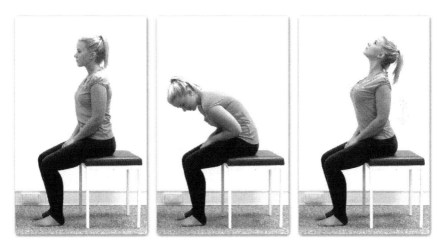

Testing in the "yes plane": neutral, bending and stretching

Test

Bend forward only as far as it is comfortable. Be mindful of the feeling when returning to the neutral position. If it is uncomfortable, you have moved too far!

When stretching you will obviously reach your movement barrier much sooner. However if you move carefully and mindfully, this could be your more comfortable direction of movement.

Once you have found out which one of the two directions is more comfortable for you, combine this movement with breathing. There are two options.

If **stretching** is the more comfortable movement for you, then breathe in while moving into the comfortable position, and breathe out while returning to the neutral position.

Now switch the breathing around: breathe out as you stretch and breathe in while returning to the neutral position. Which combination feels better? If you cannot feel a difference, pick an exercise randomly.

If your more comfortable movement is **bending forward**, then breathe in while bending forward and breathe out while returning upwards. Then the other way around: breathe out while bending forward and breathe in while returning to the neutral position. Which combination feels better?

Exercise

Repeat your "comfortable combination" of breathing and movement for several breaths. It is reasonable to take a little break after breathing in and then out, i.e. to stop breathing and movement at the same time. The length of these breaks depends on what you feel is comfortable. After a while you will better be able to feel the impulse to continue breathing.

End the exercise after two minutes. Take a short break, in which you perhaps might briefly move your shoulders or shake yourself out a little.

Retest

First test the direction of movement that you exercised. Never mind the breathing now. This movement should at least not feel worse. Now test the other direction. Can you feel a change? Normally, this movement should now feel better than it did in the initial test. If this is the case, congratulations! You have just successfully completed your first osteopathic self-treatment.

If there is no improvement or you could not feel a difference in the movements in the beginning, you probably require a different direction of exercise. The principle of the exercise, however, remains the same.

Basically, if you can feel a difference, exercise the better option. That might seem strange at first, but once you have understood it and successfully put it into practice, it becomes really easy. Sooner or later you will find an exercise after which your discomforts will suddenly disappear. From that moment on, these exercises can become highly addictive, partly because you will suddenly have the feeling that you have recovered part of the responsibility for your own health and that you can do something straight away when you feel an ache or pain.

Crucial to success is that you perform the exercises mindfully, i.e. that you put your mind and heart into the exercises.

The three planes of movement

The testing of movements is always performed on the basis of the three base planes of space, i.e. the body. The "yes plane" (sagittal plane) depicts bending and stretching movements, like e.g. nodding your head. The "no plane" (horizontal plane) depicts horizontal turning movements as e.g. performed when shaking your head. The "maybe plane" (frontal plane) depicts sideway movements, like e.g. the leaning of your head to the left and right.

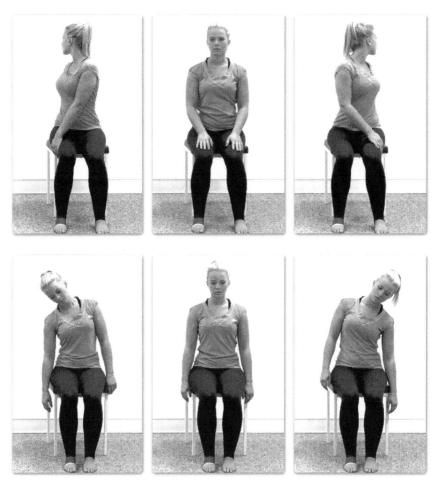

The "no plane" and the "maybe plane"

Overview of the exercise sequence

Test

Testing the movement: which is the more comfortable direction?
Testing the breathing: how does the breathing best match the more comfortable direction of movement? Does it feel more comfortable when

- you move in the better direction while breathing in and return to the middle while breathing out? Or
- when you move in the better direction while breathing out and return while breathing in?

Exercise

Repeat the "comfortable combination" of breathing and movement for several breaths or minutes. After breathing in and out, stop breathing and movement at the same time.

Retest

Retest the movement first to the better, and then to the worse side. Be aware of the difference to the initial test.

Part 1: Osteopathic Principles

Unlike you would think

When I was 17 years old I attended "Tae-Kwon-Do" martial arts classes twice a week. The training was tough and pushed me to my breaking point. And yet I never had sore muscles, except on two occasions. Due to other commitments I had to leave training early and the next day my calve muscles ached. The part of training I had missed out on, was the short meditation, sitting seiza style. In this position a large part of the calve- muscles are in maximum approximation and relaxation.

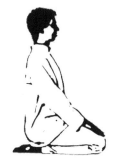

Sitting seiza-style

I did not realize at that point, that this was my first osteopathic self-treatment according to the principle of the "indirect technique", but I never forgot it.

Key principles of osteopathy

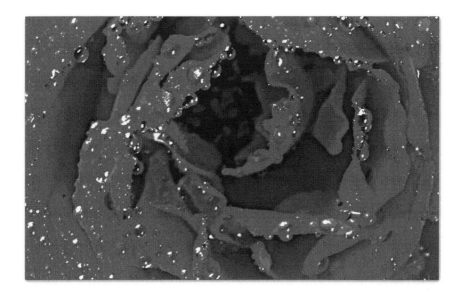

A functioning self-healing and immune system can solve virtually any health problem. Therefore osteopathy focuses on activating these oftentimes impaired self-healing powers and thereby achieve a completely natural healing.

Direct and indirect technique

In osteopathy we generally deal with two opposing directions. If we move towards a barrier, we call it the "direct technique" (directly towards the barrier). Imagine working as a waiter and carrying a dinner tray with heavy plates and glasses all day long. If you are not used to this strain, by the evening you are not able to stretch your arm properly and you feel as if your elbow were out of joint. However, if you anyway try to stretch your arm, you are working towards the barrier, i.e. with the direct technique. If you move your arm away from this barrier by bending it, so that it can relax optimally, you are applying the indirect technique. Yoga's stretching exercises correspond, from an osteopathic viewpoint, to the direct technique, whereby Yoga obviously is more than simply a stretching exercise program. Just as with all movement meditations (Qigong, Taijiquan, etc.), inner guidance of movement plays a large role with yoga and osteopathy.

The indirect technique is particularly employed in osteopathy in the case of heavy pain and large problems, because in this relieving position/direction the nourishment of the affected tissue is improved. Imagine trying to water a dry bed with a bent water hose. Moving into the position of maximum relaxation is like straightening out the bend in the hose, so that the exchange of substances can continue unhindered. In self-treatment this movement/position is mostly the more comfortable one, the "comfortable direction". To find out which one it is, you have to test both directions.

Key principles of osteopathy

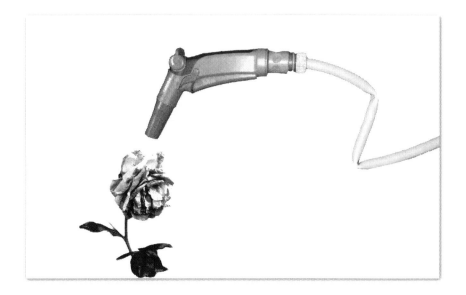

*The cause of impaired self-healing powers is a problem
with the nourishing and cleansing of the cells, the muscles,
the bones or any other structure.*

Direct and indirect technique in nature

"We believe the reason of this great absence of disease among animals and fowls of all kinds was a strict adherence to the laws under which they were placed by Nature. When they were tired the would rest, when hungry they would eat, and lived in strict obedience to all the indications of their wants. We believe man is not an exception to this rule."

A.T. Still

We can find many examples of the "indirect technique" in nature. A dog will always keep his damaged paw in a position of maximum relaxation and will lie down in a corner so that it can heal ("indirect technique"). Every now and again he will try to walk normally ("direct technique"). Once this is possible, he resumes normal walking. This is our inborn, human behavior. For example, when our stomach hurts, we bend over double, in order to allow the stomach muscles and the underlying tissue to relax optimally.

However with chronic or minor discomforts, we often suppress this natural behavior and even try to cause more tension, possibly even forcibly, along the lines of "there has to be a way!". Afterwards we wonder why our discomfort has intensified. I like to compare this behavior with a jammed door lock. Trying to open it by force will simply cause it to jam even more. However, if you gently push the lock ("indirect technique), it opens easily.

Key principles of osteopathy

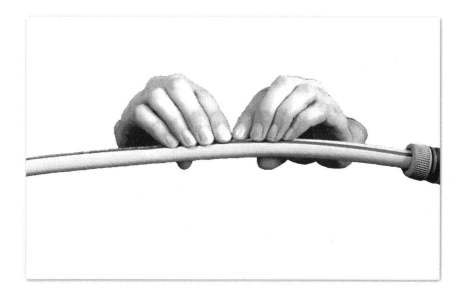

The osteopath avails himself of his profound knowledge of human anatomy and physiology, as well as finesse of his palpation to detect and do away with these problems related to nourishment and cleansing. In the case of self-treatment, your own body awareness is more than enough.

Osteopathy – supporting nature's healing powers

Dr. Still kept emphasizing, that it was the osteopath's job to find health, not illness. After all, anyone could find illness. The stance, the principle fundamental to osteopathy, is that we should focus on the aspect of "nature's healing powers". Instead of fighting illness (as a principle), we try to put the body in a position that enables healing. Try to integrate the following aspect into your thinking: when you feel ill, you already bear the seed of recovery inside yourself. This seed can grow faster, if you concentrate on your wellbeing instead of on fighting an illness.

"Activating Forces"

The conscious use of breathing is a so-called "activating force", osteopathically seen, i.e. an activating power. Activating forces make an exercise more effective, or really effective in the first place. Other activating forces are

- Emotions. You can put yourself in a certain emotional condition while performing the exercise. For example, how about closing your eyes and imagining yourself on a warm beach in the South Pacific, on a six-week holiday?

- Oscillations (vibrations). Shaking ("tou") has been known in all Qigong traditions for thousands of years. It should be used, preferably, in the breathing pauses. If you have detected on the "yes plane" that bowing your head is more comfortable than stretching it, lightly and effortlessly shake your head in the holding position.

- Stacking. All three planes of movement are adjusted one after the other, so that the maximum comfort is reached. They are "stacked". You can, e.g. test whether it is easier to turn your

25

head to the left or to the right ("no plane"), then in the comfortable position you add a small movement from the "yes plane", and finally a minimal movement from the "maybe plane". From plane to plane the movements become ever smaller, because the maneuvering room decreases.

- Own muscle strength. With some exercises you work with your own muscle strength (e.g. the exercise "pelvic area" – hip joint/pubic bone/adductors).

If you are not yet satisfied with the outcome of the exercises, simply try to employ further activating forces when performing the exercises.

Two special techniques

Not every technique is suitable for every problem, but the following two are universally useful. If they seem too complicated, simply skip this chapter.

Strain-Counterstrain (SCS)

The American physician and osteopath Dr. Jones developed the strain-counterstrain technique in the 1960s for the purpose of treating pain. It is based on the principle of wrapping tissue, i.e. the body around the painful point, as one for example does when bending over double in the case of stomach pain. The technique was slightly adapted, so that it can be used in self-treatment.

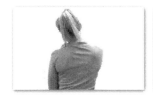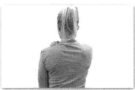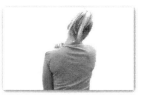

Pressure-sensitive pain points can be treated excellently with the strain-counterstrain technique

Test

If you have a point on your body that is painful under pressure, this technique is extremely useful. These are mostly found in the neck muscles. Use your right-hand fingers to find such a point on the left side of your neck.

Did you find such a pain point? Touch it so you feel a slight (!) pain in order to perform the movement tests.

Test the cervical spine on the "maybe plane". The pain probably will reduce when you tilt your head to the affected side. Leave your head like that and adjust it on the "yes-" and "no level" so that the pain possibly even disappears.

Exercise

Breathe in and out several times, consciously aware of that point, while maintaining it pain free. According to Dr Jones, it completely suffices to hold the pain point for one and a half to two minutes. Discontinue the exercise if it causes discomfort. Afterwards return to the starting position.

Retest

Take a short break, maybe shaking out your shoulders, and then retest the painful point. The pain should have reduced significantly (at least by 70%).

27

Myofascial Release (MFR)

"An intelligent head will soon learn that a soft hand and a gentle move is the hand and head that get the desired results."

A.T. Still

With MFR-techniques it is a matter of relaxing muscle and connective tissue. The hands work on the tissue. This is particularly effective with dysfunctions and pain in the muscle tissue or connective tissue (basically all pulling-related structures, such as ligaments and tendons). We have here illustrated the treatment of a painfully overstretched foot ligament due to a sprain (inversion trauma).

Test

Lightly put pressure on the affected tissue with your fingers and move it in the following directions:

- Towards your toes / towards your ankle
- Towards your lower leg / towards the sole of your foot
- Clockwise / anticlockwise

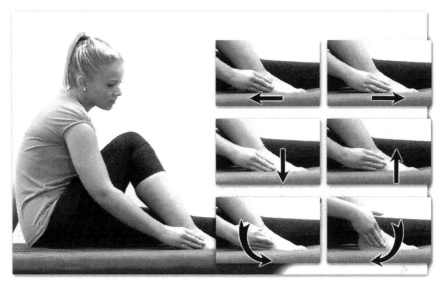

Hands on the tissue: there is always one direction that feels better than the others

Exercise

There are several exercise options:

Option A
Find the most comfortable of the six tested positions and hold the tissue there while breathing relaxed, maybe taking breathing pauses.

Option B
Again, find the most comfortable of the six tested positions. While breathing in, move the tissue into the most comfortable position, and while breathing out, return to the neutral position. Now the other way around. While breathing out, move the tissue into the most comfortable position, and while breathing in, return to the original position. Chose the more comfortable combination and repeat it for several breaths.

Option C
Stack the more comfortable directions. For example, towards the sole of your foot + towards the ankle + clockwise. Hold the tissue there. Now breathe in and out, relaxed, while holding the tissue there (as with option A).

Option D
While breathing in, take the tissue from the neutral position into the most comfortable stacked position, and hold it there for a comfortable break and return, while breathing out, into the neutral position. Then while breathing out, move into the most comfortable position and re-turn while breathing in. Chose the more comfortable combination of breathing and movement and repeat for several breaths.

Retest

Retest all movement directions. Start with the exercise movement and at the end test the worst of the six directions.

The "onion of discomfort"

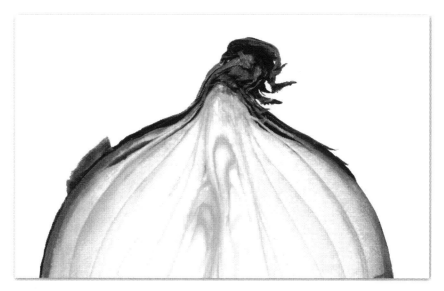

Sometimes osteopathic self-treatment is like peeling an onion

Many patients wonder why, after an osteopathic treatment of e.g. the knee, the pain in their neck is reduced. This happens all the time in osteopathy. The osteopath knows that "pain is a great liar" and therefore searches for the actual cause of discomfort.

Example: A person is in an accident and his left knee is injured. After a while this leads to often unnoticed changes in his gait. The body is constantly seeking balance (compensation). Due to its capability of compensation, e.g through the pelvis muscles, no discomfort is felt and therefore no physician is consulted. At some point another injury is sustained, maybe on the shoulder or head. Once again the body tried to balance the tensions. If the two compensations oppose each other, this causes discomfort in the neck, where two teams are playing "tug of war". The osteopath can find the trouble-causing knee or shoulder. But based on the principle of the "onion of discomfort", the patient can find the hidden cause of discomfort. In this example that means that although the neck is in pain and can therefore be called the area of the "tug of war", it is not the cause of discomfort. After a successful self-treatment of this area, the knee or shoulder will emerge as the cause of discomfort. After further self-treatment of that problem area, the discomforts should disappear permanently.

This is why osteopathy often speaks of "linkage syndrome". All the body's structures, down to the individual cell, are interlinked. We are not cars or machines made up of assembled spare parts. So it should not surprise you if discomforts wander through your body. This is often simply due to the linkage patterns of your body. If you are aware of your body and exercise it mindfully, you will soon feel that not just one particular discomfort disappears, but rather, that your movements become lighter and freer because your body's tensile stress is better distributed.

Be open to any changes that can result from the exercises, but do not expect miracles. Some discomforts disappear immediately. But you might feel a pain in another spot or you might remember something suppressed or forgotten. Clearly perceive it and decide whether it might belong to the discomfort, which lead you to perform the exercise. Your body can give you more clues to lead you to a healthier, happier life than you might think. You just need to learn to listen.

We tend to avoid taking a closer look at problems because they scare us. Fear means stress, and stress blocks the part of the vegetative nervous system responsible for healing (parasympathetic nervous system). The exercises will help you to regain your trust in nature's healing power (A.T. Still) because you no longer will be at the mercy of your discomforts. The more discomforts your have, the easier it will be for you to find the corresponding exercise, because your body gives you clear signals that something is not right.

Part 2: The osteopathic medicine cabinet

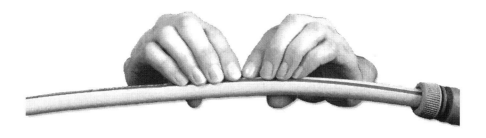

"The body of man [is] God's drug-store and [has] in it all liquids, drugs, lubricating oils, opiates, acids, and anti-acids, and every sort of drug that the wisdom of God thought necessary for human happiness and health."

A.T. Still

Dr. Still warned of a recipe-like, i.e. technical approach to osteopathy. You may adapt each exercise to your feeling. Only maintain the basic structure of "test, exercise, retest".

Note: The illustrated exercises are the result of nearly 20 years of collaboration with my patients. I was constantly searching with them for the fitting exercise and each one had to be individually adapted because no two people are the same. So I cannot promise you that "your" exercise is among these. But once you have understood the principle, you will easily find your own self-treatment options. Be playful and curious. The exercises should always be interesting and pleasant, never boring, uncomfortable or exhausting. I promise you, if you perform the exercises with awareness, you will always perceive changes.

In the words of A.T. Still,

"Now make yourself a child of inquiry and a student of Nature."

Head

Chronic Sinusitis (sinus infection)

This exercise is loosely based on an exercise developed by Dr. R.E. Becker. If you perform this exercise daily, you should notice a clear improvement after 30 days.

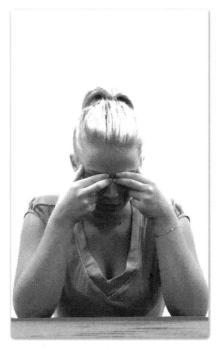

Relief in the case of chronic sinusitis

Test

First gauge the strength of your symptoms (e.g. difficulty breathing, headache, etc.)

Sit at a table and lean your elbows on it. Place the fingertips of your index and middle finger of both your hands close together at the bridge of your nose (closer to the nose than to the frontal bone). Let your thumbs rest on your temples and tuck your ring fingers and pinkies away. Test whether slightly lifting your head is better combined with breathing in or breathing out (most likely it is better combined with breathing in). While lifting your head your fingers' pressure against the bridge of your nose should slightly increase automatically.

Exercise

Repeat the better combination of breathing and movement for about 7 minutes.

Retest

Re-gauge the strength of your symptoms.

Impaired vision / eye muscles / vertigo

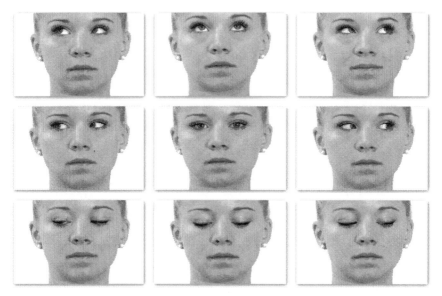

Which viewing direction feels most comfortable?

Test

Test the direction of view

- Left/right
- Upwards/downwards
- Up and to the left/up and to the right
- Down and to the left/down and to the right

If you can clearly feel which one of the eight directions of view is the most comfortable, then this is your direction of exercise. If you cannot clearly feel it, perform the exercise in the opposite direction of the least comfortable direction of view. While breathing in, look in the direction of exercise. Return to the middle while breathing out. Now the other way around. While breathing out, move your eyes in the more comfortable direction and return while breathing in.

Exercise

Perform the exercise using the option that seems easier or more comfortable. Make sure that the speed of your eye-movement matches the pace of your breathing. This requires quite some attention because you naturally move your eyes faster than you breathe. Perform this exercise for about a minute. The tension in your eye muscles changes relatively quickly, so you do not need to perform this exercise for very long.

Retest

Close your eyes for several seconds and then retest the directions of view.

Accommodation (accommodating near and far sight)

This exercise is particularly suitable for office workers working in front of a screen.

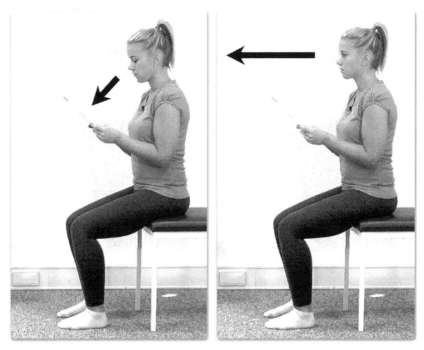

The "screen-exercise" can be performed inconspicuously at any time

Test

Focus on something at a distance of 30 to 50 cm. Then move your gaze to something in the distance (e.g. outside). Combine the more comfortable viewing distance with your breathing. Does is match better with your breathing in or out?

Exercise

Repeat the more comfortable combination of viewing and breathing for several breaths.

Retest

Retest the near- and far sight.

If this exercise does you good, repeat it frequently. It can be performed fairly inconspicuously in a large office.

Tired eyes

This exercise has Chinese roots and is known in Qigong.

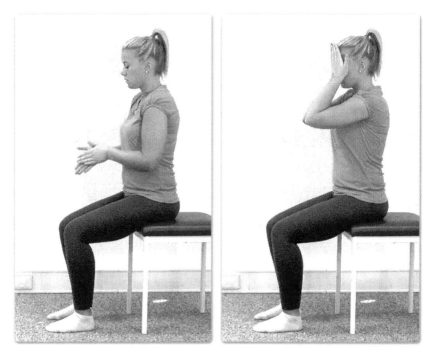

You will also find this technique in Qigong

Test

Gauge how your eyes feel.

Exercise

While breathing in and during the breathing pause, rub your hands together vigorously. While breathing out and during the breathing
pause place your hands onto your closed eyes as if you want to trans-
fer the warmth of your hands into your brain via your eyes. Repeat
this exercise at least three times.

In rare cases you might have to switch your breathing around. Just remember, the exercises are only supposed to give you an idea, which
you can adapt to your individual needs.

Retest

Gauge how your eyes feel now.

Headaches

In the case of headaches, it often makes sense to begin the treatment at your feet. You might know the proverb "Keep the head cool and the feet warm". The following exercise is particularly suitable if you are suffering of cold feet in addition to a headache. If you perform this exercise on a regular basis, you will notice a training effect: your feet will warm up ever quicker.

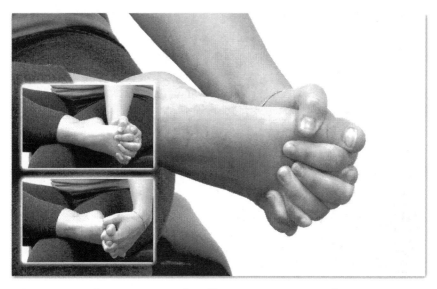

Not too easy but surprisingly effective every time: the toe exercise
Left: toes turned downwards and upwards

Test

Take your shoes and socks off and walk a few steps barefoot. Take note of the feeling in, and particularly under your feet. Now sit in a comfortable chair, although any chair will do the trick. Try grabbing your left foot with your right hand, interlinking your fingers with your toes so that your thumb and index finger are firmly grasping the big toe. Your index finger is between the big toe and the second toe. Try to stick your other fingers between your toes in the same manner.

You might have to practice this a few times. Should you not be able to stick your fingers between your toes, you can simply lay them on top and firmly grasp your foot. Is it easier to bend your toes upward or downward? Test whether the more comfortable direction is better combined with breathing in or breathing out.

Exercise

Repeat the most comfortable combination of breathing and movement for at least ten breaths. During the exercise, try to get your fingers as deep as possible between your toes in order to grasp your foot as firmly as possible. Just this once, it is okay if you feel a slight twinge.

Retest

Retest both directions and walk a few steps barefoot. You should be able to feel a clear difference in the sensation of the soles of your feet. This exercise alleviates the headache fairly quickly but your feet will probably only warm up after several hours.

Sensitive points

Patients with headaches tend to massage and rub their scalp or to press particular, sensitive points. This unsystematic, intuitively correct self-treatment can be structured.

The following exercise is based on Dr. Jones' strain-counterstrain technique.

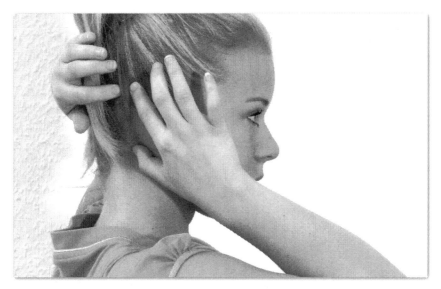

The strain-counterstrain technique performed on a pain point of the head

Test

Touch the sensitive point of your head with one finger of one hand so that you can clearly feel it. With one finger of the other hand push your scalp from one or two centimeters away towards this point.

Try to find out from which direction you have to push your scalp to clearly reduce the sensitivity. Then test the combination of breathing and movement again. Move the tissue toward the point while breathing in, and return to the original position while breathing out. Then try it the other way around and determine which way is more comfortable.

Exercise

Perform the most comfortable combination of breathing and movement for one to two minutes.

Retest

Retest the point. Its painfulness should have been clearly reduced.

Discomforts in the area of the forehead

This technique stems from the area of osteopathy that concerns itself with the skull (craniosacral osteopathy).

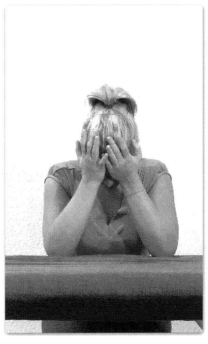

Almost a natural pose with a forehead headache

Test

Sit down at a table and comfortably rest your forehead in your hands. Now slightly turn your right underarm to the inside and at the same time your left one to the outside, then the other way around. Which is the more comfortable direction of movement? Now all you have to do, is find out which breathing phase best matches the movement.

Exercise

Perform the most comfortable combination of breathing and movement for one to three minutes.

Retest

Retest the directions of movement. If there is an improvement, the headaches will subside after a short while.

Obviously you can also perform other tests on the forehead, e.g move the hands toward and away from one another, upwards and downwards, etc.

Discomforts on the side of your head – parietal bone exercise

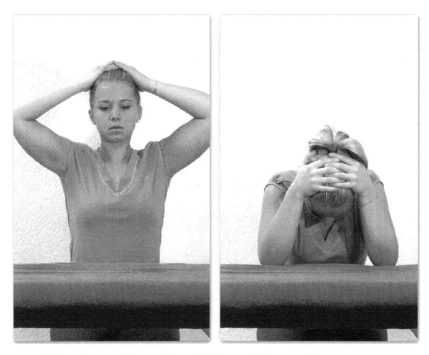

Relieving unilateral headaches, with or without support

Test

Rest your head in your hands, similarly to the previous exercise. This time, however, put some sideways pressure on the parietal bones, which you then gently pull upwards and downwards. Maintain the movement gentle, i.e. only until a slight tension is created. You can also perform this test without resting your elbows. Which direction is more comfortable? Combine it with the breathing. Is it better performed while breathing in or out?

Exercise

Perform the more comfortable combination of breathing and movement for one to two minutes.

Retest

Retest the directions of movement and check whether the worse direction has improved.

Discomforts on the side of your head – temporal bone exercise

The following exercise has an effect on the headache on the side of your head, above the temporal bones.

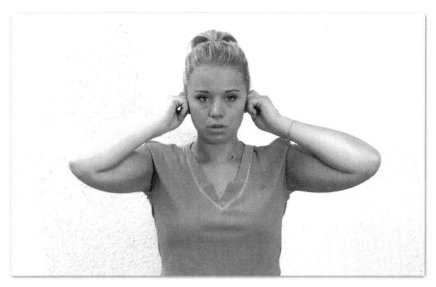

Pulling your ears to relieve headaches

Test

Grasp your ears carefully but firmly and gently pull them away from the head and forwards, and away from the head and to the back. Which is the more comfortable direction? Combine it with breathing. Is the movement better performed while breathing in or breathing out?

Exercise

Perform this more comfortable combination of breathing and movement for one to two minutes.

Retest

Retest both directions of movement and be mindful of any changes.

Options: Pull one ear up and the other one down and then switch.

If one ear is clearly more sensitive than the other, perform the exercise only with the better ear in the better direction and afterwards retest the more sensitive ear.

There are many options. Be experimental. The best exercises are often those, which you discovered yourself.

Discomforts at the back of your head

Discomforts at the back of your head often are related to dysfunctions of the upper cervical spine. So you will find the corresponding exercises in the chapter "cervical spine". The following exercise, loosely based on an exercise by Dr. Robert Fulford, can be performed sitting, standing or lying on your back.

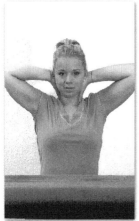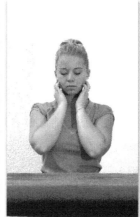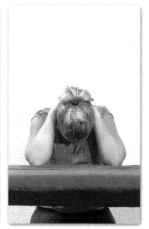

From left to right: exercise without support, feeling out the mastoid process, exercise with support

Test

Interlace your fingers and place your head in your hands so that the thenars (balls of your thumbs) touch the mastoid processes (the humps you can feel behind your ear) of the temporal bones. Gently pull the tissue of this area upwards with your thenars whilst you lower your head. Then do it the opposite way around. Lift your head and pull the tissue around the mastoid processes down. Once you have detected the more comfortable direction, combine it with breathing. Is the movement better performed while breathing in or out?

Exercise

Perform the combination of breathing and movement for one to two minutes. Be gentle and very careful. The most common mistake with this exercise is pushing or pulling too hard.

Retest

Retest both directions of movement and be aware of any changes.

Mandibular joint / teeth

Discomforts in the area of teeth and mandibular joints can have far-reaching consequences. Think of the principle of the "onion of discomfort". Here too, after successfully treating yourself, you might notice discomforts arising in other areas.

Discomforts in the jaw-area

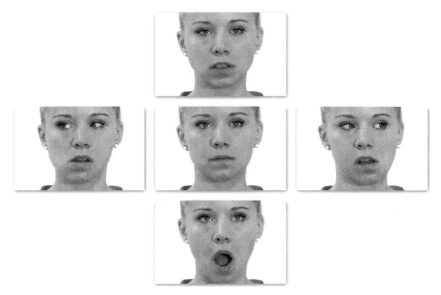

Some directions of exercise for the mandibular joint

Test

Relax your mouth open and test the following directions of movement:

Lower jaw to the right/left
Lower jaw forward/backward
Mouth opened widely/mouth closed with teeth slightly biting down on one another

Which of these six directions appears to be the most comfortable? Combine that direction with breathing. Is it performed better while breathing in or out?

Exercise

Perform that combination for one to two minutes.

Retest

Retest all six directions of movement and be aware of any changes.

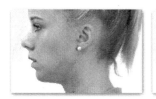 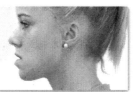 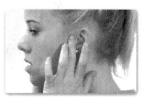

Variation: should a mandibular joint be in pain, you can place a finger on it according to the strain-counterstrain technique and press hard enough to cause a light pain. Then return your lower jaw to the most comfortable position and breathe relaxed for one to two minutes. Do not forget the breathing pauses. During the exercise, lessen the finger pressure.

Discomforts in the area of your teeth

If the cause of your discomfort is an infection, you will not notice any improvement. In that case you should visit a dentist.

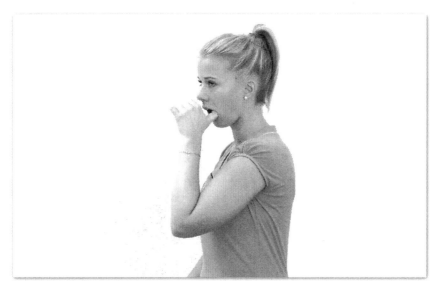

This technique can even oftentimes alleviate tooth pain

Test

Lay a finger on the chewing surface of the sensitive tooth.

Test the following options:

- Put light pressure on the tooth in direction of the back teeth/in direction of the front teeth.
- Turn your finger to the inside/outside while maintaining light pressure on the tooth.
- Put light pressure on the tooth in the direction of your lips (front teeth), cheeks (molars)/in the direction of the gums.

Which of the six directions appears to be the most comfortable? Combine that direction with breathing. Is the exercise performed best while breathing in or out?

Exercise

Perform this combination of breathing and movement for one to two minutes.

Retest

Retest all six directions of movement and be aware of any changes.

Discomforts in the throat area

If you are suffering of persistent or worsening voice problems, or difficulties swallowing, please visit a doctor. After clearing them with your physician, the presented, easily performed exercises are an excellent way to minimize your discomforts or even eliminate them.

Difficulties swallowing

Just above your voice box you will find your hyoid (tongue bone). Carefully take it between the thumb and index finger of your dominant hand.

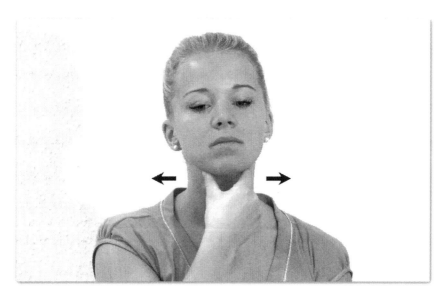

Difficulties in swallowing can be persistent and uncomfortable

Test

Move the hyoid slightly to the left/right.

Once you have found the more comfortable direction of movement, you only still need to figure out whether best to combine it with breathing in or out.

Exercise

Perform this combination of breathing and movement for one to two minutes.

Retest

Retest both directions of movement and be aware of any changes.

Should your swallowing difficulties appear at the same time as discomforts in your shoulders or arms, combine this exercise with the shoulder-arm-exercise. Your discomforts might be related to the dysfunction of a muscle connected to the hyoid via the shoulder blade.

Voice problems

For this exercise you need someone you are familiar with, who will consciously and honestly assess what he hears from you.

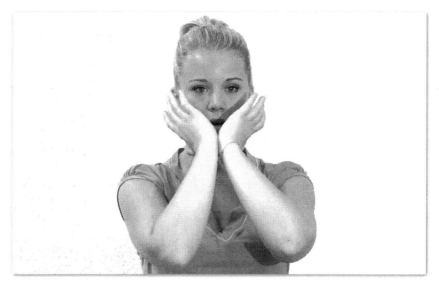

This exercise has surprising results and is worth doing on a regular basis.

Test

Sing a clearly audible, prolonged "ah" at a volume you do not yet perceive as strenuous. Let your exercise partner rate the volume on a scale of 1-10. It is helpful if he participates in the exercise, i.e. lets you rate his voice.

Exercise

Place your wrist bones together in front of your mouth, so that the tips of your middle fingers are around the area of your ears.

When you let your "ah" echo against your hands, you will notice that the sound is directed along your hands directly to your ears. You might be able to remember how it irritated you to hear a recording of your voice for the first time. We perceive our own voice differently than others do. The reason for this is that other people hear our voice through the sound that is transmitted through the air to their ear. However, we hear our voice almost exclusively through bone conduction. In this exercise the transmission of the sound over the hands lets you hear frequencies normally inaudible to you. This leads to a feedback reaction – your voice automatically becomes louder and fuller.

Sing the "ah" for as long as possible into your hands and adjust them in a way that you can hear yourself as loudly as possible. After breathing in, wait until you clearly feel the impulse to breathe out. A natural breathing and movement rhythm will set in, which you should continue for at least two minutes.

Retest

Remove your hands and sing the "ah" again. Let your partner assess the volume again. It should have increased significantly. The voice is often perceived as more pleasant or outstanding.

Spine

Cervical spine

The main exercise in cases of discomforts in the cervical spine area is performed on the "yes-", "no-" and "maybe plane".

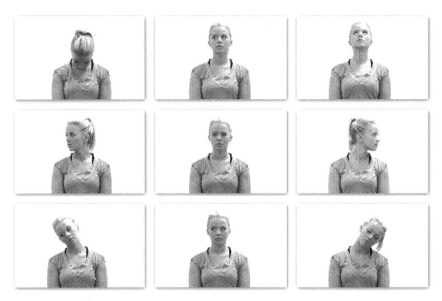

Cervical spine, "yes plane", "no plane", "maybe plane"

Test

Test which one of the following six directions of movement you perceive as most comfortable:

- Bending your head forward/stretching it back ("yes plane")
- Turning your head to the right/to the left ("no plane")
- Tilting your head towards the right shoulder/towards the left shoulder ("maybe plane")

Which of the six directions feels most comfortable? Combine it with breathing. Is the movement performed better while breathing in or out?

Exercise

Perform the most comfortable combination of breathing and movement for one to two minutes.

Retest

Retest all six directions and be aware of any changes.

For the upper cervical spine, especially in the area of the head joints, it is very useful if the movements are only minimal, as if giving a secret sign. Sometimes even just moving the eyes is sufficient.

Discomforts in the neck radiating into the head

The cervical spine is an area of pain that often stems from a completely different area. It is most important for our body to keep its eye level perfectly balanced. So if a maladjustment in the pelvic area causes the eye level to be off-balance, the cervical spine automatically compensates, which can cause discomforts. If problems keep on arising in the cervical spine area and the exercises do not provide lasting relief, note in which other body areas you sense discomfort (onion of discomfort). Applying osteopathic self-treatment to the corresponding area should reduce the discomforts in the cervical spine area as well.

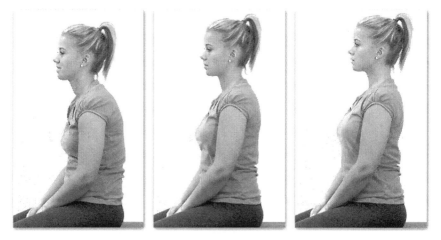

The balloon/lead-weight exercise requires some imagination

Test

Sit upright and relaxed on a chair or a stool. Make sure you have a straight posture. You might have to lift the tip of your sternum by one or two centimeters, in order to better balance your head on your cervical spine (as one would a ball on a vertical rod). Imagine your head to be light, wanting to float upwards, like a helium-filled balloon.

Now imagine your head to be as heavy as lead and your cervical spine sinking under that weight.

Test both directions without prejudice. Sometimes the "lead-head" is more comfortable, even though the "light head" sounds better.

Once you have determined the more comfortable direction, combine it with breathing. Is it better combined with breathing in or breathing out?

Exercise

Perform the combination of breathing and movement for one to two minutes.

Retest

Retest both directions of movement and be aware of any changes.

The area of the thoracic spine/chest/ribs – sitting down

Begin with the easiest exercises.

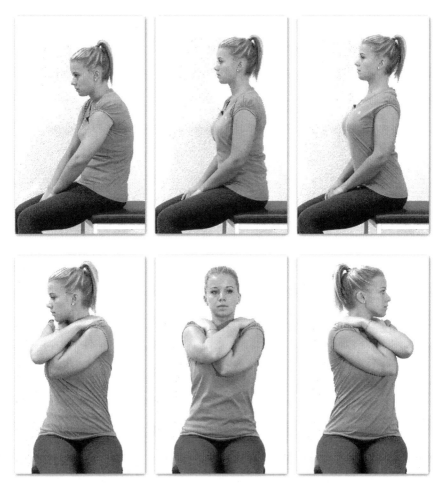

Testing the spine: above "yes plane", below "no plane"

Test

Test which one of the following six directions of movement is the most comfortable to you:

- Bending your thoracic spine forwards/ stretching it backwards ("yes plane")
- Turning the thoracic spine to the right/to the left ("no plane")
- Tilting the thoracic spine to the right/to the left ("maybe plane")

Which of the six directions is the most comfortable to you? Combine it with breathing. Is it easier to perform the movement while breathing in or out?

Exercise

Perform this combination for one to two minutes.

Retest

Retest all six directions of movement and be aware of any changes.

The area of the thoracic spine/chest/ribs – standing

The following option, performed while standing, is particularly effective. Keep your feet apart at shoulder width, your knees slightly bent. Lay your hands on the opposite shoulder and bend over slightly, so that you can feel a comfortable pull.

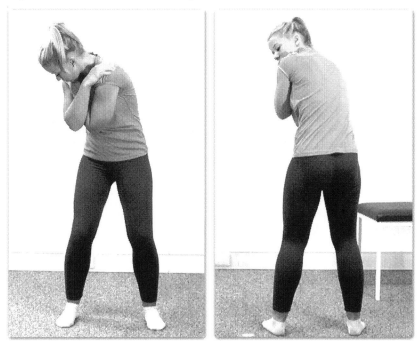

The "no plane" in a standing position

Test

Turn your torso left/right.

Have you determined the more comfortable direction? Then you just have to find out what breathing matches it best.

Exercise

Perform the combination of breathing and movement for two to three minutes.

Retest

Retest both movements and be aware of any changes.

The counterstrain exercise for the chest area

This exercise is useful e.g. for pain in the area of the thoracic spine, the ribs and the sternum. But it can also be helpful for discomforts caused by inner organs, e.g. acid reflux.

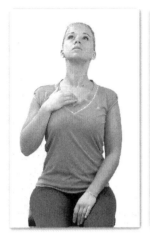
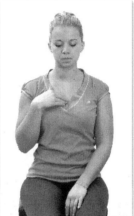
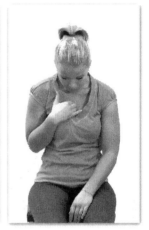

With the strain-counterstrain technique, be mindful of changes of the pain point while testing the planes

Test

Locate the pain point in the area of the sternum and the rib edges. Then test the effect of moving the spine on all three planes, one after the other. Begin by testing the bending and stretching of the upper body ("yes plane"). More often the bending leads to pain reduction. Remain in the most comfortable position. From there test on the "no plane", i.e. turn your upper body left and right and once again remain in the most comfortable position. Finally add tilting your body ("maybe plane"). The movements' amplitude keeps getting smaller with this exercise. Once you found the optimal position, the pain of the pain point should be reduced to 20% or less. The positioning of your body works best if you imagine you are wrapping yourself around the pain point.

Exercise

While maintaining the most pain free position, and holding the point with your finger, breathe in and out relaxed. Make sure that your finger pressure is gentle and not causing any pain. It might be useful to increase and decrease the pressure either while breathing in or out – try it and follow your feeling. Perform the exercise for at least two minutes. In this time you can fine-tune your position.

Retest

Slowly return to the initial position and retest the pain point. The pain should be reduced by at least 70%. Ideally you should not be able to trigger it at that point.

Exercise with stronger pain

If the pain is stronger, it is recommended to perform the exercise in a position that is as pain-free as possible. For the sternum and the lumbar spine this is often the all-fours position. You can test all three planes from this position and perform the corresponding exercise.

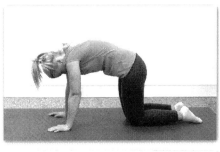

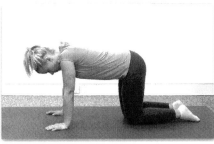

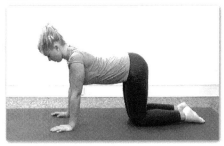

When nothing else works: the all-fours position, here the test in the "yes plane"

Test

- Bend/stretch the thoracic spine ("yes plane")
- Turn the thoracic spine to the right/to the left ("no plane")
- Tilt the thoracic spine to the right/left side ("maybe plane")

Which of the six directions feels most comfortable? Combine it with breathing. Is the movement better performed while breathing in or out?

If the movements on the "no-" and "maybe plane" are too complicated for you, simply exercise on the "yes plane".

Exercise

Perform the combination of breathing and movement for two to three minutes.

Retest

Retest the movements on the exercise plane and be aware of any changes.

Discomforts of the lumbar spine

Discomforts of the lumbar spine can often be very persistent and tend to become chronic. When asking patients how long they have suffered of these discomforts, they often answer "forever". One reason for this, that is oftentimes overlooked, is that they are not dealing with a case of limited mobility, but rather of excess mobility or instability.

The following exercises are for limited mobility.

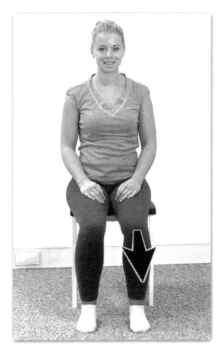

"No plane": if you push one knee forward, the pelvis turns in the corresponding direction

Test

Sit in an upright and relaxed position on a chair or a stool. Now push your right knee one to three centimeters forward, so that your pelvis begins to turn ("no plane"). Return to the original position and test the same movement with your left knee. Have you detected the more comfortable direction of movement? Now all you have to do, is find out which breathing phase best matches the movement.

Exercise

Perform the combination of breathing and movement for approximately two minutes.

Retest

Retest both movements and be aware of any changes.

While performing the exercise in the "yes plane", i.e. when bending and stretching the lumbar spine, it is helpful to imagine your pelvis being a bowl full of water. Move your pelvis as if you were carefully pouring water to the front and to the back. When tilting to the side, press one of the ischial tuberosities into the seat and imagine, viewed from the front, your lumbar spine forming a "C".

The "waves on the ocean" exercise

The Qigong exercise, "waves on the ocean", is most suitable as an additional technique following the lumbar spine exercise. It is very effective for the entire spine.

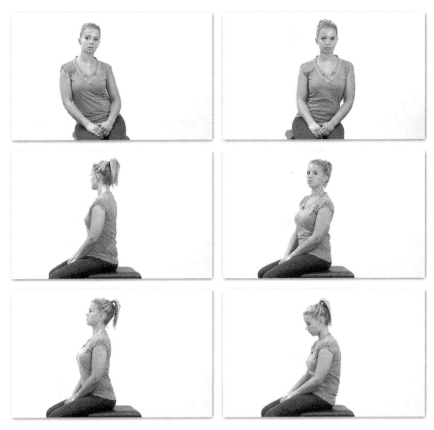

"Waves on the ocean", one of the oldest and most effective Qigong exercises

Sit in an upright and relaxed position on a chair or a stool and let your awareness sink to the lower end of your spine, to your sacral bone.

This exercise begins on the "maybe plane". Tilt your sacral bone slightly to the left (the sacral bone is just above the tailbone and below the last lumbar vertebra). Follow the spine's shifting to the left, one vertebra at a time, all the way to the head. Then you let the spine glide to the right in the same way. Do not exert yourself or try too hard. It suffices gently guiding your awareness to the area you want to move. When you repeat the movement, try to do so in an ever more fluid and faster motion. If you remain completely relaxed, you will fall into a quiet rhythm of movement that is like that of a snake. Maintain this movement until it feels smooth and your back muscles warm and loosen up.

If a particular section of your spine does not let itself be guided easily in one or the other direction, interrupt the exercise and do the following.

Test

Test whether the limited spine section can be guided comfortably in the opposite direction. If so, combine the movement with breathing. Is the movement more comfortable while breathing in or breathing out?

Exercise

Perform the combination of breathing and movement for several breaths.

Retest

Retest both directions of movement and be aware of any changes. If there is improvement, continue with the "waves on the ocean" exercise.

The "waves on the ocean" exercise can also be performed on both other planes. In the "yes plane", shift your tailbone slightly forwards. This causes the sacral bone and the entire pelvis to shift a little to the back. Then, without exerting yourself, shift all vertebrae from the bottom to the head backwards (caterpillar motion).

In the rotation ("no plane") the sacral bone and the tailbone turn together. Again, let all vertebrae follow from the bottom to the top (turning motion).

Option

In osteopathy "unwinding" refers to the untangling of the tissue. According to this technique, the self-treatment is performed as follows: After performing the exercises in the three planes separately, intuitively move out of the "no plane" into all planes simultaneously. Do this with playful ease and let yourself be guided by your feeling, as if watching your body move itself.

Unstable spine – "no plane"

Some spine problems are related to the instability of a segment of the spine. The spine has two different muscle systems: a global one, controlling all large movements of the entire body, as well as a local one, which stabilizes the spine. Imagine your spine to be a tower of building blocks or a tower of matchboxes. The global muscle system combines over large distances the bottom matchboxes with the top ones. The local system combines one box with the two neighboring ones. If something disturbs the tower's balance, the global system tenses on one side to maintain the balance. The local system, however, maintains the stability of the single segments. If there were no local system and the top and bottom box were pushed together, the boxes in between would be squashed out and the tower would collapse. The interaction of these two systems is extremely vital! The following exercises help to locate the loss of control of movement (instability) and to counteract it.

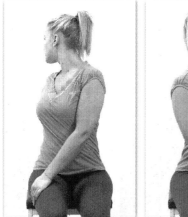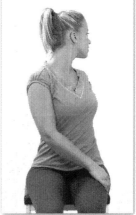

The pre-test is shown here. The actual exercise is performed without visible movements!

Test

Sit in an upright and relaxed position on a chair or a stool. Test the spine's rotation ("no plane") in both directions. While turning, be aware of the feeling in the lumbar spine and from when on the movement no longer is comfortable.

Now return to the initial position. Maintain part of your awareness in the problematic spine segment (often this is a segment of the lower lumbar spine) and imagine you are pushing your right knee forward. There should be no visible movement. The point is, that you get a feeling for controlling your muscles. You are testing the connection of your brain to your muscles. Return to the initial position and test the other knee, only in your imagination. If you can feel a distinct difference, this is probably due to a segmented instability. This might make itself noticeable by causing the feeling that many more muscles have to be utilized on one side while imagining the movement, while the other side feels like a well-functioning servomechanism. Sometimes the worse side even appears blocked. Have you detected which side is more comfortable (easier to control)? Then you just still need to find out which breathing phase best matches the movement.

Exercise

Perform the combination of breathing and movement for about two minutes. Maintain your awareness in the problematic segment. You do not require any anatomical knowledge for this. Simple feel the area. It might appear to outsiders that you have fallen asleep in a sitting position, even though, in reality, you have guided your awareness to the inside of your body and therefore are active indeed. Perform these exercises for segmented stabilization with particular inner awareness. It may take some time to obtain the desired results. Even discomforts that have existed for years have, in the case of most patients, improved after at least a month. Of course this requires daily exercise.

Retest

Retest both directions and be aware of any changes. Should it now be easier to steer towards the worse side, retest the spine's rotation like in the original test. You should perceive a significant improvement, as the two muscle systems' interaction is now more in tune.

Unstable spine – "maybe plane"

Test

Imagine you were trying to press one ischial tuberosity harder into the seat and be aware of the movement impulse. If you have instability problems, you will notice a difference when testing the other side. Which is the more comfortable direction? Which direction is easier to control? Now you only still need to match it to the right breathing phase.

Exercise

Perform the better combination of breathing and movement for approximately two minutes.

Retest

Retest and be aware of changes.

Exercise option on the "yes plane"

You should only test the "yes plane" after having done the exercises on the other planes several times or if you have so far not felt any differences.

Test

Imagine your pelvis were a bowl filled with water. Imagine you are tipping some of the water out the front. For the global muscle system, this would mean moving into an arching position, but no movement should be visible. Assess how easily you feel the impulse of movement. Now test the other direction. Imagine you are tipping some of the water out the back (causing the global muscle system to hunch your back). Test in your imagination how easily you can pull your pubic bone towards the tip of your sternum without actually moving. At the first impulse of movement in this direction you should feel your stomach muscles tensing slightly without contracting. Perform these tests playfully and without tensing up. Then assess whether one direction is easier or more comfortable than the other. Once you have decided which direction is more comfortable or easier controlled, match it to the right breathing.

Exercise

Perform the combination of breathing and movement for about two minutes.

Retest

Retest and be aware of changes

Pelvic area

Discomforts in the area of the pelvic floor

This exercise is suitable e.g. in support of a urinary incontinence therapy.

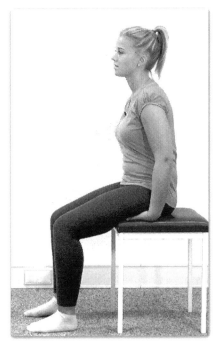

The pelvic floor exercise: gentle and effective

Test

Push the palms of your hands under your buttocks, so that the tips of your fingers can slightly grasp the ischial tuberosities.

Tense your pelvic floor. It might help imagining you are drawing your entire pelvic floor into yourself. See whether the tensing better matches breathing in or out. What counts, is the feeling of being able to control the muscles, not strength.

Exercise

Perform the combination of breathing and movement for at least two minutes. Pause your breathing for long enough to feel the inner impulse to continue breathing.

Retest

Retest you ability to control the muscles of your pelvic floor.

Discomforts in the area of the sacroiliac joint

This area is located to the left and right of the sacral bone.

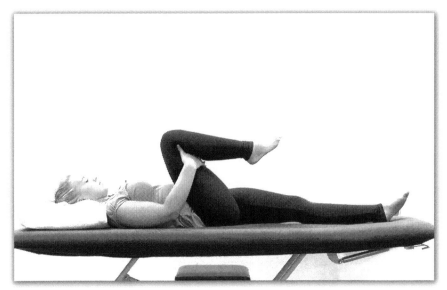

The sacroiliac joint exercise almost always has a positive effect, and often discomforts in that area are only the outer layer of the "onion of discomfort". So be mindful of any changes after the performance!

Test

Lie relaxed on a stable, but not too hard, surface. An exercise mat would be ideal. Lift your knee so far, that you can grab the hollow of your knee with your hands. If you are not able to do this, use a rolled-up towel to aid you. Be aware of how easy the movement is performed and how comfortable the final position is. Then test the other leg.

Exercise

Perform the exercise with the more comfortable side. Bend your leg and grasp the hollow of your knee with both hands.

During one breathing phase pull your leg slightly closer. During the other breathing phase move it back into the initial position. In most cases it is easier to pull the leg towards oneself while breathing in. Either way it should be completely relaxed. The movement stems from the arms and can be minimal. Perform the exercise for at least two minutes.

Retest

Retest the bending of both legs and be aware of any changes.

Discomforts in the gluteal area

The following exercise is loosely based on Dr. Johnston's "functional technique" and is wonderfully suited to the self-treatment of pain points in the gluteal area, which are often mistakenly labelled sciatica.

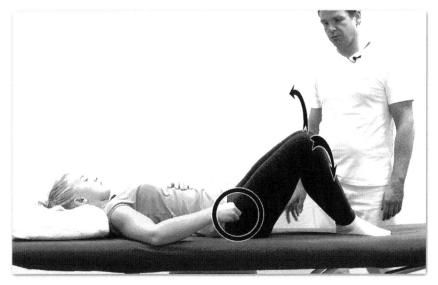

This exercise is helpful with discomforts from the gluteal area to the exterior part of the leg. It balances the pelvis.

Test

Lie on an exercise mat or on a similar surface and bend your knees with your feet remaining on the mat. Apply sufficient pressure to the pain point so that you can feel it. Hold this point and assess the tension and pain. Then slowly let the leg on the painful side fall to the outside.

Note how the tension and pain change in the point. Lift the leg back to the initial position. Now let the other leg slowly fall to the outside and take note of the pain point. Bring the leg back up to the initial position. Keep hold and take note of the point as you let both legs fall to the outside at the same time. Return to the initial position. Move both legs to the left, letting the knees and ankles touch. Afterwards move both legs to the right. One of these movements should clearly have reduced the pain and tension in the focused point. That is your exercise movement. Breathe in while moving into the more comfortable position, and out while returning to the initial position. Then switch the combination of breathing and movement, i.e breathe out while moving to the more comfortable position and breathing in while returning to the middle. Be gentle. You can often reach the most comfortable position with minimal movement.

Exercise

Perform the combination of breathing and movement with corresponding breathing pauses for several breaths.

Retest

Retest the pain point. Both pain as well as tension should be significantly reduced.

Option: During the exercise, remain in the most comfortable position and breathe in and out relaxed, not forgetting the breathing pauses.

Hip joint problems

The hip joint can be moved around all three movement axes. Usually the best results are achieved with exercises on the "no plane". You can perform the exercise lying down or standing up.

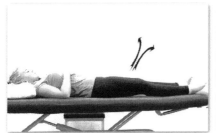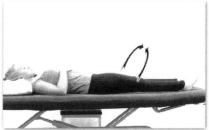

Rolling the legs to the outside and to the inside. The more gentle, the more effective!

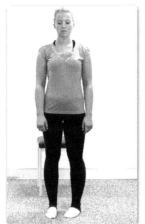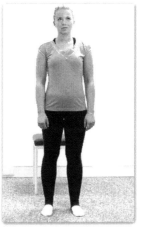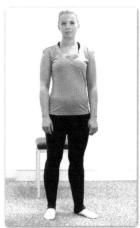

The exercise can also be performed standing

Test

Lie on your back and turn your right leg inwards/outwards. Test the left leg in the same way.

Which of the four movements is the most comfortable? Combine it with breathing. Is it best performed while breathing in or out?

Exercise

Perform the combination of breathing and movement for at least two minutes.

Retest

Retest all four directions of movement and be aware of any changes.

Option: Maintain the leg in the most comfortable position and breathe in and out relaxed. Do not forget the breathing pauses. This option is particularly suitable when performing the exercise standing up.

The area of the hip joint/pubic bone/adductors

The adductors are the muscles on your inner upper thigh. These are always tense with hip joint problems. Daily exercises over a prolonged period can be useful.

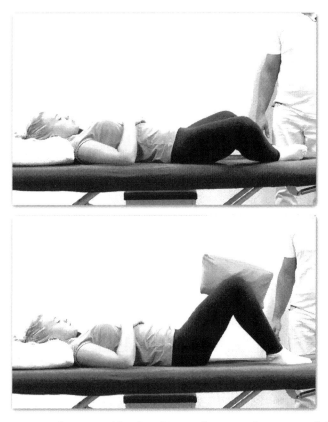

This exercise is also suitable for discomforts in the area of the pubic bone

Test

Bend your legs so that your knees create a 90-degree angle. Now slowly let your knees fall apart. As soon as you feel resistance, return to the initial position. Position your feet a little apart (30-40cm is usually the most comfortable) and press your knees together. Which position is more comfortable? If it is letting your knees fall apart then test whether it is best combined with breathing in or out. If you perceive the pressing together of the knees to be more comfortable, take a pillow or something similar, place it between your knees (the exercise can be performed without) and clasp it with your knees. Now test whether you can increase the pressure between your knees better while breathing in or while breathing out.

Exercise

Perform the most comfortable combination for at least two minutes.

Retest

Retest both options and be aware of any changes.

Knee joint

Knee exercise "healing hands"

Sit on a stable table, so that your legs hang freely off the table. Alternatively you could just sit on a chair or stool.

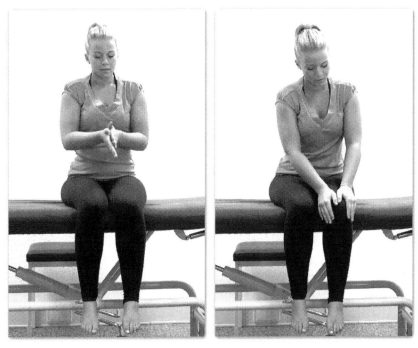

This exercise might look strange, but has proved very successful

Test

Assess the pain in your knee on a scale of 1-10.

Exercise

While breathing in and taking a breathing pause, rub your hands together vigorously so that the palms of your hands generate warmth. When you feel the inner impulse, breathe out and gently place your hands around the knee, as if you were trying to conduct the warmth of your hands into your knee. This should feel comfortable. Some prefer the opposite option - rubbing while breathing out and touching the knee while breathing in. Perform the exercise for at least 10 breaths.

Retest

Reassess the pain in your knee on the scale.

Knee exercise "turning"

Sit relaxed on a chair and place your hands, palms down, on your knees. Your feet are hip-wide apart and your ankles perpendicular to your knees.

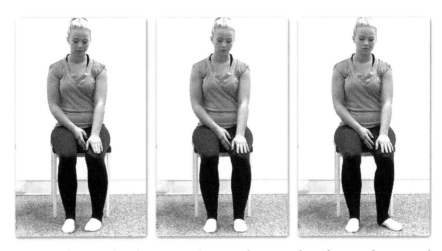

From left to right: foot turned inward, neutral and turned outward

Test

Turn your right foot to the inside. Maintain your leg's position and use your hands to stabilize your knee. Return to the initial position. Now turn your right foot to the outside. Now repeat the tests with your left foot. Which of the four directions is the most comfortable? Combine it with breathing. Does it better match breathing in or out?

Exercise

Perform the combination of breathing and movement for one to two minutes.

Retest

Retest all four directions and be aware of changes.

Exercise for the balance of the knee muscles

You need to test which of the three exercises is most effective for your knee.

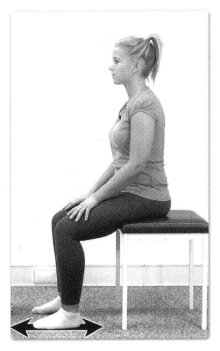

The illustrated movement is only imagined!

Test

Sit relaxed on a chair or a stool and gently press your feet into the floor. Place your hands on your upper thighs. Imagine moving your right foot forward. You will feel the muscles on the upper side of your upper thigh tense. Then imagine pulling your foot underneath the chair or stool. The muscles on the lower side of your upper thigh will tense. Which direction of tension is more comfortable? Then you only still need to find out whether it is best combined with breathing in or breathing out.

Exercise

Perform the combination for six to ten breaths.

Retest

Repeat the initial test and be aware of any changes.

Option 1: Test both legs at the same time by imagining pushing one foot away while pulling the other one under the chair or stool. Test how best you could combine breathing and tensing/relaxing your muscles.

Option 2: First test whether you can better turn your foot to the inside or to the outside and then maintain the better position. Then imagine pushing your foot away and pulling it towards you and perform the exercise with the more comfortable tension in the breathing rhythm.

Feet

You will find a good exercise for feet in the chapter titled "headaches". The following exercises are best performed lying on your back.

Problems with the upper ankle joint

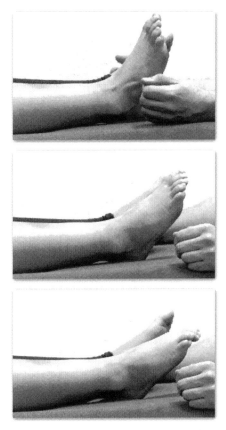

From left to right: toes pointing upward, neutral, pointing downward

Test

Test the feeling of pulling your toes towards you and stretching them away from you (movement on the "yes plane", bending/stretching in the upper ankle joint). Have you found a more comfortable direction of movement? Then you only still need to find out whether it is best combined with breathing in or breathing out.

Exercise

Perform the combination of breathing and movement for one to two minutes.

Retest

Retest both directions and be aware of changes.

Problems with the lower ankle joint

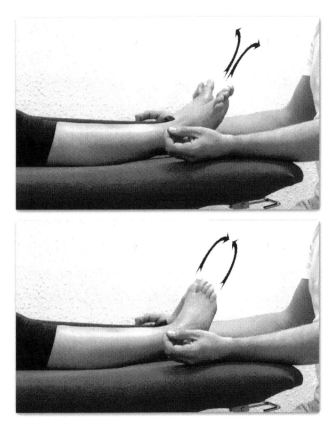

Feet turned away from each other, and the palms of the feet facing each other

Test

Test the feeling resulting from turning your ankles towards or away from one another ("maybe plane"). Have you detected a more comfortable direction of movement? Then you only still need to find out whether it is best combined with breathing in or breathing out.

Exercise

Perform the combination of breathing and movement for one to two minutes.

Retest

Retest both directions and be aware of any changes.

Sprained ankle

In the case of an acute inversion trauma ("sprained ankle"), you should set your hands to it. Bend your leg sufficiently, so that you can easily reach the injured area with your hand. Put slight pressure on the skin, so that you can feel the underlying tissue.

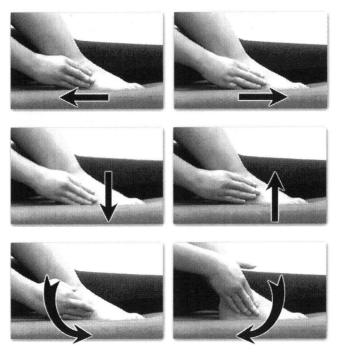

Six directions: which is the most comfortable?

Test

Move the skin and the underlying tissue in the following directions:

- Towards your pinky toe/heel
- Upward towards your knee/downwards towards the sole of your foot
- Turn the tissue clockwise/anticlockwise

Test to see how you can best match the most comfortable direction with your breathing.

While breathing in, move the tissue in the comfort direction. Hold it there while pausing your breathing. While breathing out loosen the tension and while pausing your breathing remain in the neutral position. Then try it with opposite breathing.

Exercise

Perform the most comfortable combination for one to two minutes.

Retest

Retest all six directions and be aware of any changes.

Option:
Stack the three best options. See the chapter "technique principles", MFR-technique.

Toes

Basic exercise when dealing with toe problems

This exercise is not only effective with pain in the toe joints, but also helps with cold feet.

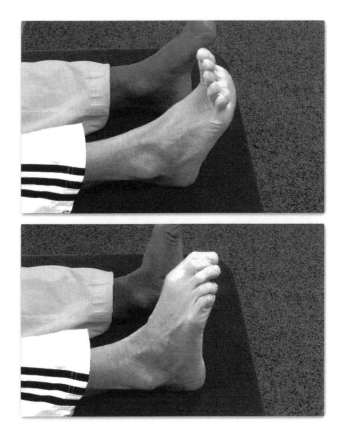

The exercise is also helpful with the tendency toward cramping. But the test movement should then only be particularly minimal.

Test

Test what it feels like to gently pull your toes towards you and stretch them away from you.

Have you found a more comfortable direction? Then you only still need to find out whether it is better combined with breathing in or breathing out.

Exercise

Perform the combination of breathing and movement for one to two minutes.

Retest

Retest both directions and be aware of any changes.

Hallux-valgus (big toe in X-position)

The following exercise can be performed sitting or lying down. It is effective against the pain and an excellent supplement to physiotherapy.

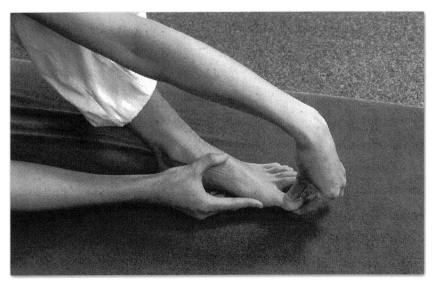

Alternatively, you can perform this exercise sitting down. It is important that you feel comfortable in the exercise position.

Test

Use a finger to search for a pain point in the area of the big toe's metacarpophalangeal joint. Hold your big toe tight with three or four fingers of your other hand and test the following eight options:

- With your fingers, bend the big toe upward/downward
- With your fingers, bend your big toe to the left/to the right
- Gently turn your big toe to the inside/to the outside.
- Gently pull your big toe to the front/push it back into the joint.

Have you found a more comfortable direction of movement? Then you only still need to find out whether it is best combined with breathing in or breathing out.

Exercise

Perform the combination of breathing and movement for one to two minutes.

Retest

Retest all eight directions and be aware of changes. The pain point should be a lot less sensitive.

Option:
Stack the more comfortable directions of the first six basic movements and hold your toe in that position. From that position, test pulling and pushing it into the joint and combine the better direction with the more comfortable breathing phase. Perform this combination of breathing and movement for one to two minutes.

Shoulders

Basic exercise for shoulder discomforts

If the following exercise does not provide any relief, try performing the next exercise for the acromioclavicular joint.

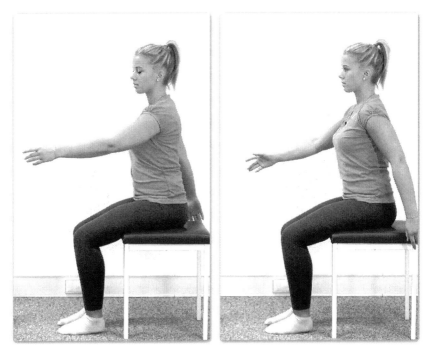

Arm movement as when walking

Test

Lift the left arm slowly, thumb pointing forward. Simultaneously, move the right arm to the back. Now the other way around: the right arm upward and the left arm to the back.

Have you found a more comfortable direction of movement? Now you only need to find out whether it is better combined with breathing in or breathing out.

Exercise

Perform the combination of breathing and movement for one to two minutes.

Retest

Retest both directions and be aware of changes.

Note: With acute discomforts, the amplitude of movement might be small. Please make sure you remain in your comfort zone.

This exercise takes place in the "yes plane". You can also perform the exercise on both other planes. On the "no plane" this means turning the affected arm to the inside/outside. One the "maybe plane" this means, stretching the arm sideways away from your body/pushing it sideways towards your body.

Dysfunctions in the area of the acromioclavicular joint

If you are suffering severe discomforts, this exercise should be performed lying on your back.

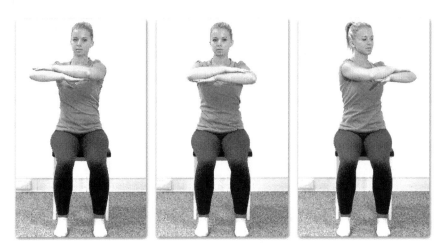

The "Kazachoc" (Cossack dance)

Test

Sit on a chair or a stool. Place your right underarm on top of your left underarm. Your chest, upper arms and underarms should form a rectangle. Without letting them break contact, move your underarms to the left. Be aware of a feeling of comfort while performing the movement, then return to the middle. Now place your left underarm on top of the right one and perform the movement to the right. Have you found a more comfortable direction of movement? Now you simply need to find out whether it is best combined with breathing in or breathing out.

Exercise

Perform the combination of breathing and movement for one to two minutes.

Retest

Retest both directions and be aware of changes.

Discomforts when lifting your arm to the front

The amount of muscle strength invested should be sufficiently low to remain comfortable.

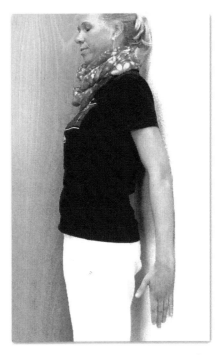

This is mostly the comfortable direction. Gently and with a lot of awareness, hold the side of your hand against the wall.

Test

Stand with your back to a wall. Let your arm hang relaxed, your thumb showing to the front. Test how far your can lift your affected arm without feeling any pain. Then test the feeling when pressing your arm slightly against the wall.

Is it comfortable? Then test whether you can increase the pressure better while breathing in or out.

Exercise

Perform this combination of breathing and pressure for one to two minutes.

Retest

Retest pressing against the wall and lifting your arm and be aware of any changes.

Option:
You can also perform this exercise lying on your back and pressing your arm into the surface you are lying on.

Note: Make sure you only apply slight pressure. If you do not notice the desired effect after the exercise, this might be due to the fact that you applied too much pressure. This is a common mistake.

Elbows

Basic exercise with discomforts of the elbows

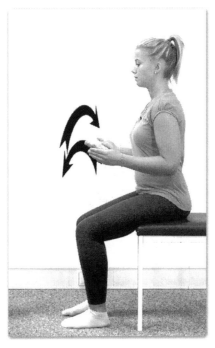

In the case of severe discomforts, you can rest the underarms on the table

Test

Sit on a chair or a stool, with your upper arms close to your body and the underarms showing forward and the thumbs upward. Test whether it is more comfortable to turn your palms upward or downward. Once you have found a more comfortable direction of movement, you only still need to find out whether it is best combined with breathing in or breathing out.

Exercise

Perform this combination of breathing and movement for one to two minutes.

Retest

Retest both directions and be aware of changes.

"Tennis elbow"

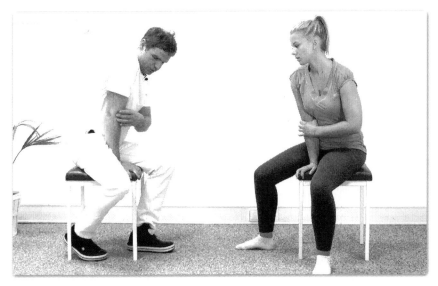

Be playful. The important thing is, that the pain is reduced significantly.

Test

Apply pressure on the pain point with one or two fingers. Rest your hand on the stool and position your arm in the most pain-free way (mostly by stretching your elbow joint). As an additional component ("activating force), add compression by moving part of your body weight onto the palm of your hand. Test whether it is more comfortable adding pressure while breathing in and reducing pressure while breathing out or the other way around.

Exercise

Perform the more comfortable combination of breathing and applying pressure for at least two minutes. The pressure should not cause any pain. Please proceed gently.

Retest

Retest the pain point. The pain should have been reduced by at least 70%.

Wrists

Basic exercise for problems in the wrist

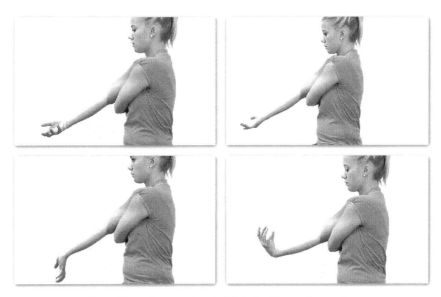

Top: Turning to the left/right from the wrist
Bottom: Bend hand downwards/pull it upwards

Test

Sit on a chair or a stool. Grab your shoulder blade under your armpit with the unaffected hand and let the arm of the affected side hang over it. The palm of your hand should be showing upward. Test the following movements:

- Pull your hand upwards/downwards.
- Move your hand from your wrist to the left/to the right.

Have you found a more comfortable direction? Then you only need to find out whether it is better combined with breathing in or breathing out.

Exercise
Perform this combination of breathing and movement for one to two minutes.

Retest
Retest all four directions and be aware of changes.

Carpal tunnel syndrome

Many of my patients managed to avoid surgery thanks to this exercise. In one case the discomforts disappeared permanently after performing the exercise once.

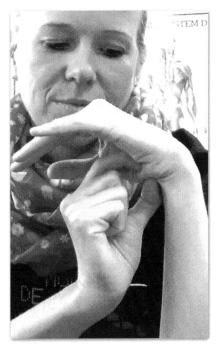

Take some time to grasp the tissue between your fingers.

Test

Sit comfortably at a table with your elbows resting on it. With the thumb and index finger of the unaffected hand, pinch the affected hand in the area between the thenar and the antithenar. Let the affected hand hang loosely so that the palm is showing downwards. With the tissue firmly fixed between your fingers, move it in the following directions:

- Towards your wrist/finger
- Towards your thenar/antithenar
- Turn it clockwise/anticlockwise

Have you detected the most comfortable direction of movement? Then you only still need to find out whether it is best combined with breathing in or breathing out.

Exercise

Perform this combination of breathing and movement for one to two minutes.

Retest

Retests all six directions and be aware of changes.

Alternative exercise "carpal tunnel syndrome"

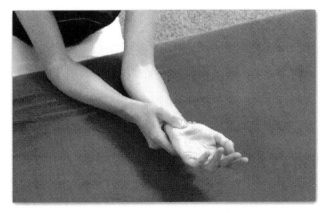

Many patients prefer this option

Test

Place the affected underarm on the table and hold your wrist so that your thumb is in the area between thenar and antithenar.

With your thumb, move the tissue as above in the following directions:

- Towards the underarm/finger
- Towards the thenar/antithenar
- Turn it clockwise/anticlockwise

Which of the six directions appears to be most comfortable? Combine it with breathing. Is it better performed while breathing in or out?

Exercise
Perform the combination of breathing and movement for one to two minutes.

Retest

Retest all six directions and be aware of changes.

Fingers

Basic exercise for fingers

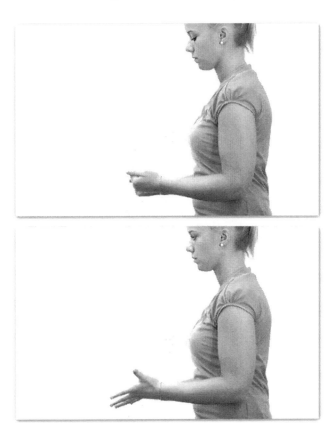

For illustrative purposes, the opening- and closing movements are amplified. The movement in the exercise, however, is a lot smaller and possibly not even visible.

Test

Close your hand into a fist and then stretch it open. What do you feel? ("sausage-finger-feeling", numbness, tension, pain, cold, etc)?

Exercise

Sit relaxed on a chair or a stool. Place your hands on your upper thighs, palms showing upward. Imagine your hands were breathing organs, like gills. Imagine them expanding as you slowly open your hands while breathing in. The movement should be barely visible. While breathing out, imagine they shrink in size, and return to the original position. Be aware of what your hands feel like. Perform this exercise for five minutes, if possible.

Retest

What do your hands feel like now? Has something changed?

The longer and the more often you perform this exercise, the faster the desired effect kicks in. I have been doing it for almost 20 years, on a regular basis, and feel marked improvement after a very short while.

For body, spirit and soul

Centering exercise

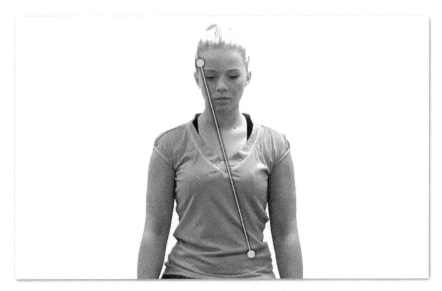

Connect the two points in your mind

Test

Test your inner balance. Stand with your feet shoulder-width apart and more or less parallel. Your knees should be minimally bent so that you can move your tailbone slightly to the front (straightening of the lumbar spine). Your spine is gently straightened; your head feels light and aims upward. In this position you feel a stronger pressure under your feet. Move your body weight onto your right foot and notice how far you can do this with ease. Then move back to the middle, pause and test the left side. Do both sides feel the same or are there differences? In the latter case, you should definitely try the following exercise.

Exercise

Remain in the position described in the test. Feet shoulder-width apart, your eyes gently closed or only slightly opened. Guide your awareness to your head. You will immediately perceive a point that draws your awareness to itself. This could be a tooth or a point on your skull, around your ear, etc. Gently take this point into your awareness and try to feel it precisely and to localize it. Where is it exactly? Now split your awareness: while being aware of the point, notice the ambient sounds (e.g. the ticking of a clock). Now guide your awareness to your body. You will straight away notice a second point. Be clearly aware of both points at the same time and in your mind connect them with a line. You could imagine this line to be a light beam, for instance. Maintain the focus of your awareness on this line and notice for several minutes what happens. If your thoughts drift, gently bring your awareness back to the line.

After some time the line appears to move towards the center of your body. But even if this does not occur, the exercise is effective. End it by stretching your knees, opening your eyes and shaking out your entire body.

Retest

Repeat the initial test and be aware of changes. How do you feel in general? Besides improving your inner balance, this exercise has a great effect on the vegetative nervous system, which among other things is also responsible for healing.

The idea for this exercise stems from a special area of osteopathy, in which we deal with "fulcrum techniques". A fulcrum is a center of rotation and pivot in the body, which the osteopath perceives with his hands. It corresponds with the line, which you could perceive in your body in this exercise. With help of the fulcrum techniques, the midline of your body is strengthened.

Exercise of the inner alchemy

"We find all of the parts of the whole solar system and the universe represented in man."

A.T. Still

The inner alchemy of antique, classic medicine deals with the training and cultivating of the spirit and psyche. The best-known exercise associated with it, is the so-called "small heavenly cycle", in which an inner movement, closely connected to your breathing, is performed. Its effect can be felt in the following exercise. At the outset of the book I asked you to notice a small stretching of your spine while breathing in. Now you will see that the opposite can happen.

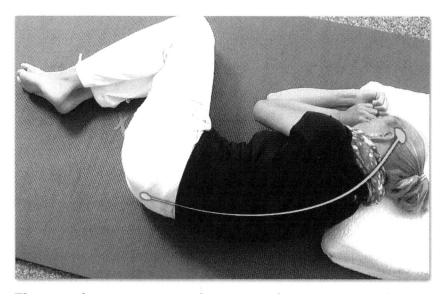

The central nervous system's key points of origin are mentally connected

Comfortably lie on your side in a fetal position. For several breaths be aware of the air flowing in and out of your nostrils. Now try to notice the air in the back of your nose, all the way into the nasopharyngeal space. Now imagine how the air travels into the area above your gums, i.e. between and behind your eyes. This is the area from which the body's central nervous system (brain and spinal cord) developed. Now place your middle- or index finger on the tip of your tailbone. Let your finger travel about 2-3 cm upward until you feel a small indentation. This is the lower end of the central nervous system. Maintain both these point in your awareness and in your mind combine them over your spine. It might help to imagine this connection as a glowing "C". When you breathe in, this "C" should bend more. When you breathe out it should straighten itself. This might be a very subtle movement, hardly noticeable from the outside. It is important that your imaginative powers remain in your body. This exercise has a strong effect on the vegetative nervous system, which means that after a few minutes you will feel very calm and relaxed.

Any questions?

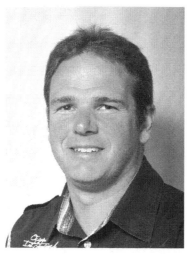

**Should you have any questions regarding the exercises,
or should you want to share experiences
or if you are interested in broadening your knowledge of osteopathic self-treatment in one of my seminars,
please visit my Facebook page:**

www.facebook.com/osteopathicselftreatment

Your Thomas Seebeck

Lotus-Press

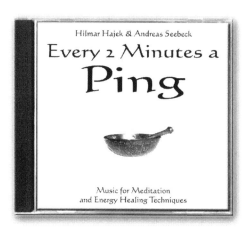

Hilmar Hajek & Andreas Seebeck

Every 2 Minutes a Ping - Music for Meditation and Energy Healing Techniques

A ping for every 2 minutes helps you to concentrate your thoughts into this healthy engagement exercise as the ping will bring your thoughts concentrated back into your meditation enabling you to take control of your mind, helping you remove those chains that binds you together with stress and depression. The music can be used to increase the effectivity for all forms of meditation practices or healing methods like Reiki, Jin Shin Jiutsu or the Healing Code. Try it now and see how effective it can be for you! Many have already tried it so why not grab that opportunity of being able to enjoy life to the fullest!

Compact Disk / mp3-download

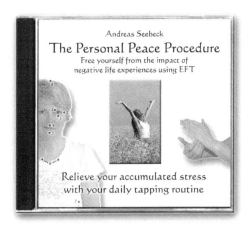

Andreas Seebeck

The Personal Peace Procedure - Free yourself from the impact of negative life experiences using EFT

Relieve your accumulated stress with your daily tapping routine.

The Personal Peace Procedure is your guide to learning the proper way on how to handle all the failures, stress and unhappy events of your life story for you to still be able to live a healthy and fit life despite the unfortunate circumstances in your life. Each of the segment is a crucial part in your healing of those hurtful feelings of the past. This procedure will help you move forward with your life and will help you see how lively it can be without weighing those negative feelings above your shoulders.

The Personal Peace Procedure uses the famous "Emotional Freedom Technique" by Gary Craig and is recommended to be done on a daily basis through identifying and resolving one problem at a time. This method has already been proven a success, so if you are one of those people who are still emotionally and psychologically distress with someone or something in the past, we recommend this method as the best way of helping you cut through those abusive ropes of misery that keeps you from seeing the beauty of what life has to offer.

Compact Disk / mp3-download

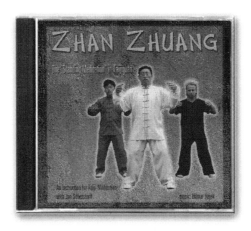

Jan Silberstorff
Zhan Zhuang

Zhan Zhuang is the Qigong exercise with the longest tradition which can be traced back 27 centuries. It is the foundation of all Qigong styles and is characterized by its great effectiveness and efficiency. For most people, training in Zhan Zhuang is a complete surprise in the beginning. There are no recognizable external movements, although it is a highly energetic exercise system. In contrast to many other methods, Zhan Zhuang develops our internal energy in a very efficient way, instead of consuming it. Zhan Zhuang Qigong is practiced in well-balanced standing positions which increase the flow of energy and build up internal strength. The Zhan Zhuang system is based on a unique fusion of relaxation and exertion which stimulates, cleanses and massages the whole body. Because Zhan Zhuang is so effective in raising our energy levels, it is often used as basic training for taijiquan.

Music: Hilmar Hajek

Tracks:
1. Instruction for beginners (22:00 min.)
2. Instruction for advanced pupils (40:00 min.)

Compact Disk / mp3-download

Made in United States
Troutdale, OR
06/19/2023

10680954R00080